NURSE MERCY

THE NURSE WITH A DIFFERENCE

MERCY UMOH

Cover Design, Book layout and Typesetting by my granddaughter NEME' Company.

ISBN: 978-978-799-253-1

Printed in Nigeria

Published by NEME Publishing Company
contact.mnumoh@gmail.com

DEDICATION

To all the nurse leaders who tirelessly strive to improve patient care and make a positive impact on the healthcare system. Your dedication, compassion, and unwavering commitment to excellence inspire us all. This book is dedicated to you.

CONTENTS

	Acknowledgments	i
	Testimonial	iii
1	A Spark Ignites	1
2	The Student Years	10
3	The First Days in White	18
4	The Heart of Nursing	27
5	A Constantly Evolving Landscape	35
6	The Challenges and Joys of Nursing	45
7	Nurses as Leaders	57
8	The Power of Resilience	68
9	Epilogue: A Life-Long Commitment	76

ACKNOWLEDGMENTS

Writing this memoir has been a deeply personal and reflective journey, but I would not have reached this point without the support and contributions of numerous individuals who have touched my life along the journey.

First and foremost, I want to express my gratitude to my family. Your unwavering love, understanding, and encouragement have been my anchor throughout this incredible journey. Thank you for standing by me, for believing in my dreams, and for being a constant source of inspiration.

To my mentors and educators, thank you for sharing your knowledge and wisdom with me. Your guidance and belief in my potential have shaped me into the nurse I am today. Your dedication to nurturing the next generation of healthcare professionals is commendable, and I am forever grateful for the impact you have had on my life.

To my colleagues, fellow nurses, and healthcare professionals, thank you for your camaraderie and support. Our shared experiences, laughter, and even tears have created an unbreakable bond. Together, we have weathered storms, celebrated victories, and upheld the highest standards of care. Your collaboration and unwavering commitment to the well-being of our patients have made a profound difference in countless lives.

To the patients and their families, I extend my deepest gratitude. You have entrusted me with your care during times of vulnerability and uncertainty. Your resilience, strength, and grace have taught me invaluable lessons and have served as a constant reminder of why I chose this path. It is an honour to be part of your healing journey.

I would also like to acknowledge the tireless efforts of the healthcare support staff, administrators, and volunteers who work behind the scenes. Your dedication and hard work ensure the smooth functioning of healthcare systems and enable us to provide the best care possible.

To the publishers, editors, and the entire team involved in bringing this memoir to life, thank you for your belief in this project. Your expertise, guidance, and commitment to excellence have been instrumental in shaping this book.

Lastly, I want to express my heartfelt appreciation to the readers—those who have chosen to embark on this journey with me. Your interest and openness to the stories and experiences shared within these pages mean the world to me. It is my sincere hope that this memoir serves as a source of inspiration, encouragement, and understanding, fostering a deeper appreciation for the nursing profession.

While the acknowledgments listed here are but a glimpse of the many individuals who have influenced and supported me throughout my nursing career, please know that every person I have encountered has played a role in shaping the nurse and person I am today.

With deepest gratitude,

Mercy Umoh.

TESTIMONIAL

Testimony about Mrs. Mercy Nseobong Umoh, By Mrs. Mary Nathan (nee Mary Elijah Awah), Retired Nurse Practitioner and Educator (RGN, RMHN, RNT, MSc, Dip HE), UK

Mercy has been my childhood friend since the 1950s when I was in primary school. I have always seen her as my role model and elder sister, because I do not have an elder biological sister. Mercy and her biological family have been very significant in my life. There is no dimension of my life that her family has not impacted, whether professional, spiritual, marital, or social. In personality, Mercy is a very hardworking and focused lady. These are among the qualities I admire about her, even as a young person then. She is very committed and treats everything with a business attitude. She plays when it is necessary, but she occupies most of her time with serious attention.

Because of how Mercy behaved and presented herself, I wanted to pattern my life after hers, to do everything that would make me productive and helpful to the family and to others. I wanted to go to the same secondary school that she went to, at Cornelia Connelly College (CCC), Afaha Oku, Uyo. I was admitted in 1961, but because of financial constraint, I could not attend the same secondary school with her. It was painful to me because I thought if I did not go to the same school as she, maybe I would not become as good as she was. But I took it that it was not God's will for me to go to the same school. When she finished school, she wanted to be a nurse, so I also wanted to be a nurse. She studied nursing in Ibadan, and I also wanted to do my own nursing in the same University College Hospital (UCH) Ibadan. Again, this did not turn out to be, but I went on to do my own nursing training in another hospital. After her nursing qualification in Nigeria, Mercy moved to the UK to continue her nursing practice and education. She got married and in early 1980s she returned to Nigeria with her husband and children. In January 1990, I was admitted continuing my nursing education and practice in the UK. I worked there since then till I retired in December 2013.

Mercy and I have continued to keep in touch, in our professional, family, and spiritual lives, and how we could be of help to our families and to other people, and how to shine out our light as Christians. With my professional life, she has been a great influence, and a constant mentor and motivator in other areas of my life. At the family front, Mercy's father had two wives and the second wife (after Mercy's mother) was my first cousin, Late Mrs. Margaret George Utuk (aka Nne Maggie). I got closer to her family because of my relationship with her. It was from there I became close to the children of my cousin (Nee Margaret Esenam Akpan Awah).

In my marriage, Mercy's elder stepbrother, Elder Sunny George Utuk represented my family at my wedding in Kaduna, in December 1972. He gave me out at the wedding ceremony: when the officiating minister asked, "who gave this woman to be married to this man", he responded, "I am". So, Mercy was directly and indirectly connected with my marital life. Her younger brother, Dr. Nseobong George Utuk, also travelled all the way from Akwa Ibom State (then part of South-eastern State) to attend my wedding in Kaduna. He is an American citizen currently living in the USA and is a Minister of the Gospel of the Lord Jesus Christ, Mercy could not attend my wedding because she was living in the UK at that time, but her two brothers were there for me.

For my spiritual life, Mercy’s elder brother, Elder Edet George Utuk had spoken to me about Jesus Christ as Lord and Saviour in the early 1960s. But I did not fully understand then, and I did not pray to receive Christ at that time. Elder Edet Utuk played a significant role in my educational advancement as he gave me inspiring counsel towards my desire and pursuit of nursing education. He also gave me remarkable spiritual support and encouragement when my husband sought my hand in marriage.

It was Mercy's younger brother Dr. Nseobong George Utuk that gave me a Gospel tract that I read, and I accepted Jesus Christ as my Lord and Saviour on 18th June 1970. The tract was titled "How can ye escape the damnation of hell?" (Matthew 23:33b), by Oswald J Smith, the founder of Peoples Church in Toronto, Canada. I was particularly captivated by scripture references as 1 Corinthians 6:9-10; Romans 3:23; Romans 6:23; James 2:10; Ephesians 2:8-9; and John 14:6. It became clear to me what it means to be a Christian, that it is not just about going to church or doing church activities but seeing myself as a sinner who could not save myself, and accepting the Lord Jesus as the Substitute and Redeemer who died for my sin. I learnt that if I believed, I would then become a child of God and the Lord Jesus would be my Saviour. It was on that day that I got to understand that salvation and escaping going to hell is by grace alone, through faith alone, and in Christ alone. Moreover, Dr. Nseobong George Utuk has maintained regular support in my Christian walk.

On one occasion, when I needed a legal service, Mercy's first daughter, Mrs. Ofonimeh Abudu, a legal practitioner and British citizen, who lives and practises in the UK, provided me with a free legal service, which sufficiently brought positive outcome. At Ofonimeh's degree Law school graduation at University of Newcastle, UK, my husband attended but I couldn't because of my official commitment. Three of our adult children and I attended her wedding, also in Newcastle.

Daniel, our son, attended and graduated from the same university as Samuel Imayak, Mercy's son. Samuel was in his final year at Bryan College, Dayton, Tennessee, USA, when Daniel was in his first year. He confirms that his own traits of hard work, positive skills, and commitment were further reinforced by Samuel's support.

So, Mercy has had much impact in the professional, spiritual, and marital aspects of my life. In my life generally, I am a serious-minded person - whatever I need to do, I want to do it with all my heart. That is one of the virtues I learnt from Mercy. She is a very committed and contented born again Christian. She is very focused and supportive. She is very resilient: things that break other people down can hardly break Mercy down, because of her commitment to the Lord Jesus Christ.

I pray that Mercy will enjoy many more years of God's abundant grace and excellent walk with our Lord and Saviour Jesus Christ. Mercy and I pray that everyone who reads this piece will accept Christ Jesus as their personal Lord and Saviour, and thus escape going to hell.

PREFACE

As I sit down to write this memoir, I am overwhelmed with a profound sense of gratitude and purpose. Nursing has been woven into the very fabric of my being—a vocation that has shaped my life in immeasurable ways. It has granted me the privilege of witnessing humanity's vulnerabilities and triumphs, the honour of being present during moments of both sorrow and celebration.

In the following pages, I embark on a journey to share the depths of my experiences as a nurse—a journey filled with countless stories that have left an indelible mark on my heart. Whether you are someone contemplating a career in nursing, a seasoned professional seeking solace in shared experiences, or an individual whose life has been touched by the compassion of a nurse, this memoir is dedicated to you.

To the aspiring nurse, I offer guidance and inspiration, shedding light on the winding path that awaits you. The road may be demanding, but it is also filled with rewards beyond measure. You will bear witness to the beauty of the human spirit and find purpose in moments that others may overlook. My hope is that my stories will ignite the flame within you, encouraging you to take up this noble calling with unwavering determination and compassion.

To my fellow nurses, my comrades in arms, this memoir serves as a tribute to our shared experiences—the long hours, the emotional toll, and the relentless pursuit of excellence. It is a reminder that we are not alone, that our struggles and triumphs are part of a collective tapestry that binds us together. May these pages bring comfort, validation, and a renewed sense of purpose to your tireless efforts in the face of adversity.

And to those who have been on the receiving end of a nurse's care, this memoir seeks to honour your journey and illuminate the immense impact nurses have on the lives of their patients. It is a testament to the unwavering commitment and empathy that nurses bring to their practice. Through my stories, I hope to capture the essence of the nurse-patient relationship—the delicate balance between technical expertise and heartfelt connection that makes nursing an art as much as it is a science.

This memoir is not just my story; it reflects the collective experiences, struggles, and triumphs of countless nurses who have dedicated their lives to caring for others. It is a celebration of the resilience, dedication, and unwavering spirit that defines our profession.

As we embark on this journey together, I invite you to open your heart and mind, to walk in the shoes of a nurse, and to witness the profound beauty and complexity of our world. Through the highs and lows, the tears and laughter, I hope that the pages of this memoir resonate with you, inspire you, and remind you of the incredible power that lies within each one of us to make a difference.

With love and gratitude,

Mercy Umoh.

1

A SPARK IGNITES

It all started with a spark. A moment in my childhood that ignited a fire within me—a fire that would eventually guide me towards a career in nursing. In this chapter, I share the experiences that inspired me to pursue nursing, as well as the challenges I faced in my journey to become a nurse.

It all started with a spark. A flicker of destiny that would shape the course of my life—a calling that would lead me down the noble path of nursing. In this chapter, I share the experiences that ignited the flame within me, the challenges I faced, and the unwavering motivation that propelled me towards becoming a nurse.

As a young girl growing up in Nigeria, I was surrounded by a bustling household, filled with the laughter and love of my family. But it was during a time of adversity that I discovered the true essence of compassion and the profound impact it could have on others.

I vividly remember an outbreak of influenza in 1957 that swept through our community, leaving countless families in its wake. Amidst the chaos, my own household became a battleground against this unseen enemy. I watched as my sister, her husband, and the children under our care succumbed to the illness, their strength diminishing day by day. I became their caregiver, their lifeline in a time of desperation.

In those tender moments, I witnessed the transformative power of care and empathy. With each soothing touch, every tender word, I saw hope flicker in their eyes. It was as if my presence alone had the ability to ease their pain, to bring a glimmer of comfort to their suffering souls. It was in those moments of nurturing, as I wiped away tears and held their hands, that I realized the tremendous impact a nurse could have on the lives of others.

Years later, as I stood in the hallowed halls of Cornelia Connelly College, I continued to cultivate my nurturing spirit. Assigned the responsibility of maintaining cleanliness within the school, I embraced my duties with an unwavering commitment. Each day, I swept through the corridors, ensuring that the classrooms were spotless, the school hall was inviting, and the newly constructed science block gleamed with potential.

But it was one fateful day, as time seemed to slip through my fingers like grains of sand, that I faced a challenge. Overwhelmed by my workload, I reached out to a fellow student for assistance. As the moments ticked away, I hurriedly checked her progress, only to find that she had overlooked the science lab—a crucial aspect of our responsibilities.

Frantic and determined not to let down the faculty, I rushed to rectify the oversight. And in the flurry of my haste, tragedy struck. My arm, desperate to fulfil its duty, found itself caught in the sharp embrace of the window blades. The pain was searing, and crimson rivulets of blood painted my arm—a testament to my unwavering dedication.

It was in that moment, as I trembled with pain and uncertainty, that the true resolve within me awakened. I realized that nursing was not merely a profession—it was a calling that demanded unwavering commitment, resilience in the face of adversity, and a heart willing to bear the weight of others' suffering. The scars on my arm served as a tangible reminder of the sacrifices I was willing to make to bring solace and healing to those in need.

But the journey towards becoming a nurse was not without its trials. As I found myself in the sterile confines of the hospital, seeking treatment for my injury, I encountered a nurse who personified the very opposite of the care I aspired to provide. Her impatience and lack of empathy etched themselves into my memory, a stark contrast to the tenderness I had hoped for. In that moment, my resolve solidified I would be a nurse who would shatter these callous stereotypes, a beacon of compassion in a world that often seemed devoid of it.

It was there, in that hospital room, amidst the echoes of my sister's untimely demise and the sting of the nurse's indifference, that I made a solemn vow. I would dedicate my life to nursing, to becoming a nurse who would embody empathy, kindness, and unwavering support for those entrusted to my care. No patient would ever be left feeling helpless or alone in their moments of vulnerability.

And so, with purpose burning brightly within me, I embarked on a path that would test my limits, challenge my resilience, and nurture my spirit. Little did I know that this spark, born from adversity and fuelled by compassion, would guide me through a lifetime of service and define the very essence of who I am.

To those who yearn to become nurses, let my story be a testament that the journey is not for the faint of heart. It demands sacrifice, unwavering determination, and a passion for uplifting others in their darkest hours. To my fellow nurses, may my experiences serve as a reminder of the impact we have on the lives of those we serve—a reminder that our care extends far beyond the physical realm and into the depths of the human spirit. And to the retiring nurses who have dedicated their lives to this noble profession, may my words resonate with the bittersweet nostalgia of a journey well-travelled, and the knowledge that your legacy lives on in the hearts of those you have touched.

In the chapters that follow, I invite you to walk alongside me, as we explore the triumphs, the challenges, and the extraordinary beauty that exists within the world of nursing. Together, let us embrace our calling, nurture the flickering flames within our souls, and ignite a fire of compassion that will forever illuminate the path we tread. For in nursing, we find not only our purpose, but a profound connection to the hearts and lives of those we serve.

REFLECTIVE THOUGHTS

1. **Exploring Your Calling:** Reflect on the experiences and moments in your life that have ignited your desire to become a nurse. What specific events or encounters have shaped your understanding of the nursing profession? How do these experiences align with your core values and purpose? Consider how your calling to nursing can fuel your motivation and commitment to serving others.

2. **Nurturing Empathy and Compassion**: Reflect on the significance of empathy and compassion in nursing. How do you define these qualities, and how do you envision incorporating them into your interactions with patients and their families? Explore ways to cultivate empathy and compassion in your own life, such as seeking to understand others' perspectives or engaging in acts of kindness and service.

3. **Embracing Challenges and Resilience:** Reflect on the challenges and obstacles you may encounter on your journey to becoming a nurse. How do you perceive these challenges as opportunities for personal growth and

resilience? Identify specific strategies or mindset shifts that can help you navigate and overcome adversity in pursuit of your nursing goals.

4. **Building a Supportive Network:** Reflect on the importance of a strong support system in your nursing journey. Who are the individuals or communities that can provide guidance, encouragement, and mentorship? Consider how you can actively seek out and engage with supportive networks, such as joining nursing associations or connecting with experienced nurses, to enhance your learning and professional development.

5. **Crafting Your Unique** Nursing Identity: Reflect on what kind of nurse you aspire to be. How do you envision making a difference in the lives of your patients? Consider the values, qualities, and skills you want to embody as a nurse and how you can cultivate them. Reflect on how your personal experiences, strengths, and unique perspective can shape your nursing identity and contribute to the holistic care of your patients.

These reflective prompts encourage self-exploration

and introspection, helping individuals who desire to become nurses delve deeper into their motivations, values, and aspirations. Through reflection, they can gain clarity, strengthen their commitment, and cultivate the personal growth necessary to embark on a fulfilling nursing journey.

Actions for Mentoring Future Generation Nurses

1. **Foster a passion for nursing:** Share your own passion for nursing with aspiring nurses. Talk about the rewards and fulfilment that come from the profession. Encourage them to explore their own motivations and aspirations, helping them develop a deep-rooted passion for nursing.

2. **Provide guidance on educational pathways:** Guide future nurses through the educational requirements and options available to them. Share information about nursing programs, prerequisites, and different educational pathways such as associate degree programs, bachelor's degrees, or accelerated programs. Offer insights on choosing the right program that aligns with their goals and interests.

3. **Mentorship through shadowing and clinical experiences:** Offer opportunities for aspiring nurses to shadow you or other experienced nurses. Allow them to observe your daily work and clinical interactions, providing them with first-hand experience of what it's like to be a nurse. Support them

during clinical rotations by providing guidance, answering questions, and offering constructive feedback.

4. **Share practical tips for success:** Draw from your own experiences and provide practical tips and advice for success in the nursing profession. Discuss effective study techniques, time management skills, and strategies for navigating the challenges of nursing school and clinical practice. Encourage them to develop good communication skills, critical thinking abilities, and professionalism.

5. **Instil the values of compassion and empathy:** Emphasize the importance of compassion and empathy in nursing. Discuss the impact of showing kindness and understanding to patients, families, and colleagues. Encourage future nurses to develop their interpersonal skills and to cultivate a patient-centred approach to care.

By mentoring future generation nurses, you can help shape their understanding of the profession, guide them through their educational journey, and install the values and skills necessary for success and compassionate care. Your mentorship can play a significant role in inspiring and supporting their growth as they embark on their own nursing careers.

2

THE STUDENT YEARS

The journey of becoming a nurse is far from easy. This chapter delves into my experiences as a nursing student—learning the ropes, building relationships with peers and mentors, and facing the inevitable challenges that come with balancing academic demands and personal life.

As I stepped onto the campus of the University College Hospital (UCH) in Ibadan, I couldn't help but feel a tingle of excitement mixed with nervous anticipation. The hallways echoed with the footsteps of fellow nursing students, their conversations brimming with enthusiasm and a shared commitment to make a difference in the world of healthcare. Little did we know that the next few years would shape us in ways we never imagined.

In those hallowed halls, the classrooms became our sanctuaries of knowledge. We were introduced to a world of medical jargon, complex concepts, and the art of nursing. Anatomy and physiology textbooks soon became our closest companions, their pages dog-eared and filled with scribbled notes as we delved deeper into the intricacies of the human body.

But nursing education was not confined to lectures alone. It was in the clinical rotations that the lessons truly came alive. Stepping onto the wards for the first time, dressed in our pristine white uniforms, we were a mix of excitement and trepidation. The scent of disinfectant mingled with the sounds of beeping machines and hurried footsteps, creating a symphony unique to the hospital environment.

Under the watchful eyes of experienced nurses, we embarked on a journey of hands-on learning. From assisting with patient care to administering medications, we were given opportunities to apply our theoretical knowledge in real-life situations. There were moments of awe and wonder as we witnessed the birth of a new life, and moments of heartache as we comforted grieving families. Each patient interaction left an indelible mark on our souls, reminding us of the privilege and responsibility inherent in the nursing profession.

As nursing students, we relied not only on textbooks and clinical instructors but also on each other for support and camaraderie. We formed study groups that met late into the night, pouring over complex medical cases, and dissecting the intricacies of nursing care plans. These moments of collaboration not only deepened our understanding of the material but also forged lifelong friendships and bonds that would carry us through the challenges ahead.

Yet, the student years were not without their fair share of hurdles. The workload was relentless, demanding long hours of study, sleepless nights, and endless assignments. There were days when exhaustion threatened to engulf us, when doubts whispered in our ears, questioning our capabilities.

But it was during those moments that we found solace in the unwavering support of our peers, who reminded us of our resilience and the passion that burned within us.

Life, too, continued to unfold amidst the chaos of our studies. Relationships bloomed, some faltered, and life outside the hospital walls demanded attention. I remember the struggle of balancing the demands of my nursing education with the responsibilities of being a partner, a parent, a friend. There were times when guilt tugged at my heartstrings, wondering if I was neglecting those, I held dear. But in those moments, I realized that by pursuing my calling, I was not only enriching my own life but also becoming a role model for my loved ones—a testament to the importance of pursuing our passions fearlessly.

The student years were a time of transformation. We evolved from eager novices to budding professionals, equipped with a deep understanding of patient care, critical thinking skills, and the resilience required to navigate the healthcare landscape. We embraced the challenges head-on, learning to adapt, to think on our feet, and to thrive in an environment where lives hung in the balance.

Yet, it wasn't just the academic and clinical aspects that shaped us. It was the stories of patients we encountered, the laughter and tears shared with fellow students, and the wisdom passed down by experienced nurses that left an indelible mark on our hearts. We witnessed the triumph of the human spirit, the fragility of life, and the power of compassion in healing not just physical ailments, but also emotional wounds.

As the student years ended, we stood on the precipice of a new chapter—a chapter that would see us donning the title of registered nurses, ready to make our mark on the world. With a mixture of excitement and apprehension, we embraced the unknown, armed with the knowledge that our education had prepared us well for the challenges and joys that lay ahead.

Looking back, I am grateful for the student years—the lessons learned, the friendships forged, and the unyielding determination that carried us through. The University College Hospital became more than just an institution—it became a crucible that transformed us into nursing professionals driven by compassion, dedicated to the well-being of our patients, and resilient in the face of adversity.

The student years were not just a means to an end; they were a formative chapter in the tapestry of my nursing career. They laid the foundation upon which I would build my future, shaping not only my clinical skills but also the core values that would guide me throughout my professional journey. The student years were the catalyst that ignited my passion for nursing, forever imprinting upon my soul the belief that the care we provide can truly change lives.

And so, with a mix of nostalgia and anticipation, I closed the door on the student years, ready to step into the world as a nurse—a humble guardian of health, an advocate for patients, and a lifelong learner in the pursuit of excellence. The path ahead was unknown, but I was armed with the knowledge that my education had prepared me well, and that the student years were just the beginning of an extraordinary adventure.

REFLECTIVE THOUGHTS

1. What were the most memorable moments from my nursing student years? Reflect on specific experiences, challenges, or accomplishments that stood out to you during this period.

2. How did the academic demands and clinical rotations shape my understanding of nursing? Consider the knowledge and skills you acquired and how they contributed to your growth as a future nurse.

3. What were the most significant lessons I learned from my clinical instructors and mentors? Reflect on their guidance, teachings, and the impact they had on your development as a compassionate and competent nurse.

4. How did I navigate the balance between my nursing education and personal life during this time? Explore the challenges you faced in managing your time, responsibilities, and relationships, and reflect on the strategies you used to maintain equilibrium.

5. How did my experiences as a nursing student influence my perception of the nursing profession? Consider how your interactions with patients, colleagues, and the healthcare system shaped your understanding of the role and impact of nurses in healthcare.

Remember, journaling is a personal and reflective practice, so feel free to delve deeper into these questions, exploring your emotions, insights, and personal growth throughout your nursing student years.

Actions for Mentoring Future Generation Nurses

1. **Share your experiences and stories:** One of the most valuable ways to mentor future generation nurses is by sharing your own experiences and stories from your nursing career. By recounting both the challenges and the triumphs you've encountered, you can provide valuable insights and guidance to aspiring nurses.

2. **Provide guidance on career paths and specializations:** Nursing offers a diverse range of career paths and specializations. As a mentor, you can help future nurses navigate these options by providing information about different specialties, advanced practice roles, and opportunities for growth. Discuss the pros and cons of each path and offer advice based on your own experiences.

3. **Offer advice on educational and professional development:** Guide aspiring nurses on the educational and professional development opportunities available to them. Share information about relevant certifications, advanced degrees, and

continuing education programs that can enhance their knowledge and skills. Help them develop a plan for their professional growth and offer resources or connections that may assist them in achieving their goals.

4. **Teach the importance of self-care and resilience:** Nursing can be emotionally and physically demanding, and it's crucial to instil the importance of self-care and resilience in future nurses. Share strategies for maintaining a healthy work-life balance, managing stress, and seeking support when needed. Encourage them to prioritize their own well-being to ensure longevity and fulfilment in their nursing careers.

5. **Foster a culture of collaboration and continuous learning:** Emphasize the value of teamwork, collaboration, and lifelong learning in the nursing profession. Encourage future nurses to seek opportunities for interdisciplinary collaboration, engage in professional organizations, and stay updated on the latest research and advancements in healthcare. Inspire them to be curious, open-minded, and committed to delivering the best

possible care to their patients.

By serving as a mentor and sharing your knowledge, experiences, and guidance, you can help shape the next generation of nurses, empowering them to thrive in their careers and make a positive impact in the lives of their patients and communities.

3

THE FIRST DAYS IN UNIFORM

After years of hard work, I finally graduated and embarked on my career as a registered nurse. In this chapter, I share my initial experiences as a new nurse, discussing the excitement, nervousness, and the overwhelming sense of responsibility that comes with this role.

The day had finally arrived—the day I would step foot into the hospital as a registered nurse. The anticipation and excitement were palpable as I walked through the sterile corridors, dressed in my pristine white uniform. The weight of the responsibility I was about to undertake settled upon my shoulders, mixing with a nervous flutter in my stomach.

Entering the nursing station, I was greeted by the bustling atmosphere of dedicated healthcare professionals. The scent of disinfectant and the gentle hum of medical equipment filled the air, creating a unique ambiance that I would soon become intimately familiar with. Nurses in their experienced white uniforms moved with purpose and grace, their knowledge and expertise evident in their every action.

I was assigned to a senior nurse who would be my mentor during those initial days. Her warm smile and reassuring demeanour eased my nerves as she guided me through the labyrinthine halls of the hospital. The mentorship program was designed to provide support and guidance to new nurses, helping us acclimate to the demands of the profession.

My first days as a nurse were a whirlwind of orientation, training, and shadowing experienced nurses. I was introduced to the intricacies of patient charting, medication administration, and the various protocols that governed every aspect of our care. Each day brought new challenges and opportunities to learn, as I observed and assisted in different procedures, from dressing wounds to administering injections.

While the classroom had prepared me with theoretical knowledge, the true essence of nursing came alive within the patient rooms. It was here that I encountered individuals at their most vulnerable, facing illness, pain, and uncertainty. I witnessed first-hand the immense impact a nurse could have on their well-being, not only through medical interventions but also through a compassionate touch, a listening ear, and a comforting presence.

I vividly remember my first patient encounter—an elderly woman who had just undergone surgery. Her frailty was apparent, and her eyes held a mixture of fear and hope. As I introduced myself and explained the care plan, I could feel the weight of her trust in me. It was a humbling experience, a reminder of the profound responsibility we carry as nurses to uphold the highest standards of care and empathy.

In those early days, I immersed myself in the art

of nursing. I learned to read the subtle cues and expressions of patients, deciphering their needs beyond the confines of medical charts. I discovered the power of a gentle touch or a comforting word, realizing that sometimes, providing solace to a worried patient could be as vital as administering medication. The white uniform I wore became more than just a symbol of professionalism; it became a tangible representation of the trust bestowed upon me by those in need.

As the days turned into weeks and the weeks into months, I grew more confident in my abilities. The white uniform that once felt foreign and pristine became a garment that held within it the countless stories of patients I had cared for. It became a symbol of my dedication and commitment, a badge of honour that reminded me of the privilege it was to serve as a nurse.

The first days in white were filled with moments of joy, tears, and triumphs. I celebrated the small victories—the successful administration of medications, the smiles and gratitude from patients, and the camaraderie among the nursing staff. And yet, there were moments of doubt, when the weight of responsibility felt overwhelming, and I questioned whether I had what it took to make a difference in the lives of those entrusted to my care.

But through it all, I learned that nursing is not a solitary journey. It is a collective effort, a harmonious symphony of healthcare professionals working together to improve the lives of their patients. I forged bonds with fellow nurses, forming a support network that uplifted me during the most challenging times and celebrated my achievements alongside me.

The first days in white were a transformative period—an initiation into a world where compassion, dedication, and resilience were the guiding forces. I emerged from those days with a deeper understanding of the immense privilege it is to be a nurse. The journey had just begun, and I was eager to continue growing, learning, and making a difference—one patient at a time.

As I reflect upon those early experiences, I recognize that the first days in white were not only about becoming a nurse but also about discovering the nurse within myself. It was a journey of self-discovery, as I learned to navigate the complexities of human emotions, cultivate empathy, and find strength in moments of vulnerability.

The first days in white were a beautiful initiation into the world of nursing—a world where compassion and expertise intertwine, where small gestures can bring comfort, and where the connection forged between a nurse and a patient can create profound impact. With each passing day, I continue to honour the privilege of wearing white, striving to make a positive difference in the lives of those I have the honour to care for.

REFLECTIVE THOUGHTS

1. **Embracing the Responsibility:** The first days in white taught me the weight of the responsibility that comes with being a nurse. It is a privilege to be entrusted with the care of patients during their most vulnerable moments. Embracing this responsibility requires a deep commitment to providing the best possible care and advocating for the well-being of those we serve.

2. **The Power of Compassion:** Nursing is not just about medical interventions and treatments; it is about compassionately connecting with patients on a human level. The first days in white showed me the profound impact a simple act of kindness or a listening ear can have on a patient's well-being. Compassion has the power to heal, uplift spirits, and bring comfort during times of distress.

3. **The Value of Teamwork:** Nursing is a collaborative profession, and the first days in white taught me the importance of working as part of a team. The support and guidance from experienced nurses and the camaraderie among fellow nurses became invaluable sources of

strength and knowledge. Together, we could provide comprehensive care and navigate the challenges that arose with greater efficacy.

4. **Balancing Confidence and Humility:** The transition from a student to a registered nurse can be both exciting and overwhelming. While gaining confidence in our skills and knowledge is essential, it is equally important to maintain humility. Recognizing that there is always more to learn and being open to new experiences and perspectives allows us to continuously grow as nurses.

5. **The Beauty of Connection:** Nursing is a profession that fosters meaningful connections between caregivers and patients. The first days in white highlighted the beauty of these connections—the ability to create trust, provide comfort, and make a positive impact on someone's life. These connections remind us of the human element in healthcare and the significance of empathy in our interactions.

These reflections from my first days in white continue to shape my approach to nursing. They remind me of the privilege and responsibility that comes with wearing the uniform, and they inspire me to continuously strive for excellence in the care I provide. The lessons learned in those early moments have become the foundation upon which I build my career as a nurse—a career fuelled by compassion, dedication, and an unwavering commitment to the well-being of others.

Actions for Mentoring Future Generation Nurses

1. **Share Personal Experiences:** As a mentor, you can provide valuable insights by sharing your own experiences as a nurse. Talk about the challenges you faced, the lessons you learned, and the rewarding moments that made it all worthwhile. By sharing your journey, you can inspire and motivate future nurses, helping them navigate their own paths.

2. **Offer Guidance on Building Skills:** Mentoring involves helping aspiring nurses develop the necessary skills to excel in their profession. Provide guidance on areas such as critical thinking, communication, time management, and decision-making. Offer practical tips and advice based on your own experiences and encourage them to seek out opportunities for growth and skill development.

3. **Foster a Supportive Environment:** Create a safe and supportive space for future nurses to ask questions, seek guidance, and share their concerns. Let them know that you are there to support them throughout their journey. Encourage open and honest communication and be a compassionate listener when they face

challenges or need someone to talk to.

4. **Promote Continuous Learning:** Nursing is a field that is constantly evolving, with new research, technologies, and practices emerging regularly. Encourage the future generation of nurses to prioritize lifelong learning and professional development. Recommend resources, workshops, conferences, and online courses that can enhance their knowledge and skills. Instil in them the importance of staying updated and adapting to changes in healthcare.

5. **Lead by Example:** Be a role model for aspiring nurses by demonstrating professionalism, compassion, and integrity in your own practice. Show them what it means to be a dedicated nurse who puts the well-being of patients first. Model effective communication, teamwork, and empathy in your interactions with colleagues and patients. Your actions and attitudes will serve as powerful lessons for those who look up to you.

Remember, mentoring is not only about providing guidance but also about nurturing the next generation of nurses to become confident, compassionate, and skilled healthcare professionals. By sharing your knowledge, experiences, and support, you can make a lasting impact on their professional journeys.

4

THE HEART OF NURSING

At the core of nursing is the ability to provide compassionate care to patients and their families. In this chapter, I share some of the most memorable and inspiring patient encounters that have left a lasting impact on my life, shaping my understanding of what it means to be a nurse.

At the core of nursing is the ability to provide compassionate care to patients and their families. It is within the intimate moments of vulnerability and the connections we form that the true essence of nursing shines through. In this chapter, I delve into some of the most memorable and inspiring patient encounters that have left a lasting impact on my life, shaping my understanding of what it truly means to be a nurse.

Each day as a nurse brings new challenges and opportunities to connect with patients on a profound level. I vividly recall an encounter with a patient who had been admitted to the hospital's emergency ward with a severe case of difficulty passing urine. The patient was in agonizing pain, and their family anxiously awaited the arrival of a male nurse, believing that only a male caregiver could address their needs. However, as the only available nurse at that moment, I found myself faced with a difficult decision.

Approaching the family with empathy and understanding, I explained the situation, assuring them that I would do everything within my power to provide the necessary care. Though their consent was initially hesitant, they entrusted me with their loved one's well-being. With a prayer for strength and a heart filled with determination, I embarked on the procedure. It demanded a delicate balance of technical expertise and emotional support as I worked to alleviate the patient's suffering.

As the treatment progressed, I could feel the tension in the room slowly dissipating. The patient's pain subsided, and a sense of relief washed over them. It was a powerful reminder of the immense trust patients place in nurses and the profound impact we can have on their lives, even in the most challenging circumstances. The family, once apprehensive, expressed gratitude for the care and compassion I had shown, recognizing that it was not the gender of the caregiver but the dedication and expertise that truly mattered.

Another significant patient encounter remains etched in my memory—an incident that unfolded while I was off duty but happened to be present at the hospital. A patient was being admitted with difficulties passing urine, and the attending nurse urgently sought my guidance.

Drawing upon my knowledge and experience, I swiftly assessed the situation and provided instructions to the nurse. Together, we created an environment that encouraged relaxation and the natural flow of urine. Placing a warm towel on the patient's belly, just above the pubis, and preparing containers for collection, we offered comfort and support. As the sound of water cascaded from the kettle into the waiting container, a sense of calm enveloped the room, and the patient experienced a renewed sense of ease.

This encounter underscored the fact that nursing transcends the confines of time and duty. It reminded me of the importance of being ever ready, physically, and mentally, to lend a helping hand whenever and wherever it is needed. As nurses, we hold the responsibility of making a positive difference in the lives of those we care for, and sometimes that means going above and beyond our designated roles.

These stories, among countless others, exemplify the heart of nursing—a profound commitment to alleviate suffering and provide comfort to those in need. We have the privilege of being present during some of the most intimate and challenging moments in a person's life, allowing us to witness their strength, vulnerability, and resilience. It is through our compassion, empathy, and unwavering dedication that we create a healing environment, foster trust, and instil hope in our patients and their families.

In the upcoming chapter, I will delve into the ever-evolving landscape of nursing, exploring the diverse roles and settings nurses can embrace. Additionally, I will emphasize the significance of lifelong learning and professional development in this noble profession, as we strive to provide the highest quality of care and continue to grow as compassionate healthcare providers.

REFLECTIVE THOUGHTS

1. **Compassion:** The experiences I've shared in this chapter highlight the power of compassion in nursing. It is not just about providing medical care but also about being there for patients and their families during their most vulnerable moments. It's about offering a listening ear, a comforting touch, and a reassuring smile. These small gestures can make a significant difference in the healing process.

2. **Building Relationships:** Nursing is more than just a series of tasks; it's about building meaningful connections with patients. The stories I've shared demonstrate the importance of taking the time to understand their fears, hopes, and dreams. By forming genuine relationships, we can provide holistic care that addresses not only their physical needs but also their emotional and spiritual well-being.

3. **Resilience:** Nursing can be emotionally challenging, and it requires resilience. The encounters I've described in this chapter involved patients in pain, families in distress,

and moments of uncertainty. It is through resilience that we find the strength to keep going, to advocate for our patients, and to provide quality care even in the face of adversity.

4. **Empathy:** Empathy lies at the heart of nursing. Putting ourselves in our patients' shoes allows us to better understand their experiences, fears, and concerns. The stories shared in this chapter demonstrate the impact of empathy on patient outcomes and the healing process. It is through empathy that we can truly connect with our patients and make a difference in their lives.

5. **The Joy of Nursing:** Despite the challenges, nursing brings immense joy and fulfilment. The moments of connection, the gratitude of patients and their families, and the knowledge that we have made a positive impact in someone's life are the rewards that keep us going. The stories I've shared reflect the profound joy that comes from being a nurse and being able to touch lives every day.

Actions for Mentoring Future Generation Nurses

1. **Foster Empathy:** Encourage aspiring nurses to develop their empathetic skills. Help them understand the importance of seeing patients as individuals with unique stories, experiences, and emotions. Encourage them to actively listen, observe body language, and respond with genuine care.

2. **Teach Communication Skills:** Effective communication is vital in nursing. Help future nurses develop strong communication skills, including active listening, clear and concise verbal communication, and the ability to provide information in a compassionate manner. Emphasize the importance of non-verbal communication and building trust with patients.

3. **Highlight the Value of Teamwork:** Nursing is a collaborative profession, and teamwork plays a crucial role in providing comprehensive care. Encourage future nurses to value and respect the contributions of their colleagues, foster a supportive team environment, and communicate effectively

within the healthcare team.

4. **Promote Self-Care:** Nursing can be demanding both physically and emotionally. Teach aspiring nurses the importance of self-care to prevent burnout and maintain their own well-being. Encourage them to establish healthy boundaries, seek support when needed, and engage in activities that promote self-care and work-life balance.

5. **Instil a Lifelong Learning Mindset:** Nursing is an ever-evolving field, and it is important to instil a passion for lifelong learning in future nurses. Encourage them to stay updated with advancements in healthcare, pursue professional development opportunities, and seek out mentorship from experienced nurses to continuously grow and improve their skills.

By reflecting on the heart of nursing and mentoring future generation nurses, we can ensure that the spirit of compassion, dedication, and resilience.

5

A CONSTANTLY EVOLVING LANDSCAPE

The world of nursing is ever-changing, and as a nurse, it is essential to adapt and grow. In this chapter, I discuss my journey through various nursing roles, specializations, and settings, highlighting the importance of lifelong learning and professional development.

The world of nursing is ever-changing, and as a nurse, it is essential to adapt and grow. In this chapter, I discuss my journey through various nursing roles, specializations, and settings, highlighting the importance of lifelong learning and professional development.

Throughout my career as a nurse, I have had the privilege of working in a diverse range of roles and settings. Each experience has been a steppingstone in my professional growth, teaching me valuable lessons and expanding my understanding of the nursing profession.

After completing my initial training at the esteemed University College Teaching Hospital of Ibadan, I was given the opportunity to lead the general nursing department in the outpatient department. As the sole nurse in the department, I faced the challenge of learning on the job. This experience not only sharpened my clinical skills but also instilled in me a sense of responsibility and resilience. I quickly learned to adapt to the demands of providing quality care with limited resources. It was during this time that I truly grasped the significance of effective time management, critical thinking, and empathetic communication with patients.

Seeking to further enhance my knowledge and skills, I pursued additional education in the field of midwifery at Deborah Maternity Hospital in the United Kingdom. This intensive training provided me with a comprehensive understanding of prenatal, childbirth, and postnatal care. I learned to support expectant mothers through the various stages of pregnancy and deliver safe and compassionate care during childbirth. The experience exposed me to the vulnerability and joy associated with bringing new life into the world. As a midwife, I developed a profound appreciation for the importance of building trust, providing emotional support, and promoting maternal and infant well-being.

Although my journey as a midwife was rewarding, I felt a deep desire to explore other specializations within nursing. I decided to embark on specialized training in the field of special care nursing for infants. This experience exposed me to the delicate nature of neonatal care and the challenges faced by premature or critically ill infants. Through this training, I gained knowledge in the areas of developmental care, monitoring vital signs, and providing specialized interventions. I witnessed the strength and resilience of these tiny patients and their families, as well as the dedication required to ensure their well-being. It reinforced the importance of collaboration with a multidisciplinary team and staying up to date with advancements in neonatal care practices.

Motivated by a commitment to occupational health and safety, I pursued further education in occupational health nursing. This specialized field allowed me to work closely with employees in various industries, focusing on preventing work-related illnesses and injuries. I learned to conduct comprehensive assessments of work environments, identify potential hazards, and implement proactive measures to promote a healthy and safe workplace. As an occupational health nurse, I collaborated with employers and employees to develop effective health promotion programs, educate about ergonomics and personal protective equipment, and provide timely interventions for occupational health issues. It was a role that emphasized the importance of prevention, education, and ongoing monitoring to create a healthy work environment.

Throughout my career, I embraced opportunities for professional growth and development. One such opportunity was the role of a clinical nurse tutor, where I had the privilege of guiding and inspiring the next generation of nurses. This role allowed me to share my knowledge and experiences, while also cultivating my own teaching and leadership skills. I discovered the power of mentorship and the immense satisfaction that comes from seeing students grow and flourish in their nursing journeys. It reinforced the importance of supporting the future of nursing through education and fostering a culture of lifelong learning.

Returning to Nigeria, I sought new challenges and opportunities to contribute to healthcare in different settings. I worked in various hospitals, including the fast-paced emergency department, where I served as a head nurse. This dynamic environment demanded quick thinking, effective decision-making, and the ability to provide immediate care to those in critical situations. It was a humbling experience, as I witnessed the impact of teamwork, clear communication, and the importance of continuous professional development to keep up with the latest advancements in emergency care.

In 1990, I joined the Midwives Service Scheme (MSS), a non-profit organization focused on reducing maternal and infant mortality rates.

This experience took me to Tofa Local Government Area, Kano Region, where I worked tirelessly to provide comprehensive maternal and child healthcare services to underserved communities. Through the MSS, I witnessed first-hand the power of community engagement, health education, and early interventions in improving health outcomes. It reinforced my belief that nursing goes beyond the bedside and extends into the communities we serve. It emphasized the significance of culturally sensitive care, health advocacy, and the impact nurses can have in transforming lives at a population level.

As I reflect on my journey through various nursing roles and settings, one thing remains clear nursing is a constantly evolving profession. From advancements in technology and research to changing healthcare policies and practices, nurses must continuously adapt and update their knowledge and skills. Lifelong learning is not just a choice; it is an essential part of being an effective and compassionate nurse.

To aspiring nurses, I encourage you to embrace the evolving landscape of nursing. Be open to new opportunities, seek out specialized training, and never stop learning. Embrace challenges as opportunities for growth and remember that the impact you can have on the lives of patients and their families is immeasurable.

To my fellow nurses, continue to be the advocates and change-makers in the healthcare system. Embrace collaboration, mentorship, and lifelong learning to provide the best possible care to those who rely on us.

And to those who work with nurses—patients, families, and healthcare colleagues—understand the dedication, expertise, and compassion that nurses bring to their roles. Support their ongoing professional development and acknowledge the pivotal role they play in the healthcare ecosystem.

As I conclude this chapter, I am filled with gratitude for the ever-evolving landscape of nursing that has shaped me into the nurse I am today. It is a privilege to be part of a profession that touches lives, promotes healing, and embodies the essence of humanity. Through continual growth and adaptation, we can continue to make a meaningful difference in the lives of those we serve.

REFLECTIVE THOUGHTS

1. **Lifelong learning is essential:** Throughout Chapter 5, I emphasize the importance of continuous learning and professional development in the nursing field. Each new role and specialization I pursued required me to acquire new knowledge and skills. This journey reinforced the notion that nursing is a constantly evolving profession, and staying abreast of advancements is crucial to providing high-quality care. Reflecting on this, I am grateful for the opportunities I had to expand my expertise and contribute to the well-being of patients.

2. **Adaptability is key:** As I transitioned through different nursing roles and settings, I realized the significance of adaptability. Whether it was learning on the job as the sole nurse in a department or embracing a new specialization, being adaptable allowed me to navigate challenges effectively. Nursing demands the ability to adjust quickly to varying situations and environments, and through my experiences, I developed a resilient mindset that helped me thrive in

ever-changing circumstances.

3. **Collaboration drives success:** Chapter 5 highlights the power of collaboration within the nursing profession. From working alongside multidisciplinary teams in neonatal care to partnering with employers in occupational health, I witnessed first-hand how teamwork enhances patient outcomes and promotes a healthy work environment. Reflecting on this, I value the relationships I formed with colleagues and the collective effort that goes into providing holistic care.

4. **Nursing extends beyond the bedside:** While my journey encompassed diverse nursing roles, one common theme emerged nursing goes beyond the bedside. Through my involvement with the Midwives Service Scheme and community outreach programs, I experienced the transformative impact of nursing at a population level. It reinforced the understanding that as nurses, we can influence health outcomes beyond individual patients, shaping policies and advocating for better healthcare access for all.

5. **The privilege of making a difference:** Reflecting on my journey, I am reminded of the privilege that comes with being a nurse. The ability to contribute to the well-being of individuals and communities is a profound honour. From assisting in childbirth to providing emergency care and advocating for improved healthcare, every interaction and opportunity to make a positive impact has been a humbling experience. This reflection reinforces my dedication to the nursing profession and the ongoing pursuit of excellence in patient care.

Actions for Mentoring Future Generation Nurses

1. **Foster a culture of mentorship:** Actively participate in mentoring programs and initiatives within your healthcare organization or community. Offer guidance, support, and advice to aspiring nurses and those in the early stages of their careers. Encourage a culture where experienced nurses are eager to share their knowledge and help shape the next generation of nursing professionals.

2. **Share personal experiences:** Reflect on your own nursing journey and share your personal experiences with aspiring nurses. Discuss the challenges you faced, the lessons you learned, and the moments that inspired you. By sharing your stories, you can provide valuable insights and encouragement to those who are just starting out in their nursing careers.

3. **Provide learning opportunities:** Create opportunities for hands-on learning and skill development. Offer shadowing experiences, allow mentees to observe and participate in various nursing procedures, and provide guidance in critical thinking and decision-

making. Encourage mentees to take advantage of educational resources, workshops, and conferences that can enhance their professional growth.

4. **Encourage self-reflection and goal setting:** Help mentees develop self-awareness and encourage them to reflect on their strengths, areas for improvement, and long-term goals. Assist them in setting achievable objectives and creating action plans to work towards their aspirations. Regularly revisit these goals and offer guidance and support to keep them motivated and on track.

5. **Promote continuous professional development:** Emphasize the importance of lifelong learning and ongoing professional development. Encourage mentees to pursue specialized training, attend seminars or webinars, and stay updated with the latest research and advancements in nursing practice. Provide guidance on professional organizations and resources that can support their growth and help them navigate opportunities for further education and certifications.

By taking these actions, you can contribute to the development and success of future generations of nurses. Through mentorship, you have the power to inspire, guide, and shape the next wave of nursing professionals, ultimately strengthening the nursing profession.

6

THE CHALLENGES AND JOYS OF NURSING

Nursing, like any profession, comes with its fair share of challenges. This chapter delves into the emotional, physical, and mental trials that I have faced as a nurse and the ways in which I have learned to cope with them.

Nursing, like any profession, comes with its fair share of challenges. This chapter delves into the emotional, physical, and mental trials that I have faced as a nurse and the ways in which I have learned to cope with them.

Every day in the life of a nurse presents unique challenges that test our mettle and resilience. The long hours, demanding schedules, and emotionally charged situations can take a toll on even the most dedicated and passionate caregivers. However, it is in these moments of adversity that we find the strength to persevere and the true joys of nursing.

One of the greatest challenges I have faced as a nurse is witnessing the pain and suffering of my patients. I have held the hands of individuals battling chronic illnesses, comforted grieving families, and walked alongside patients facing their darkest moments. Each experience has taught me the importance of empathy and compassion in providing holistic care. Despite the emotional weight that accompanies these encounters, I have found solace in knowing that I can offer comfort and support to those who need it most.

Nursing also demands physical stamina and resilience. The physical demands of the profession can be gruelling, with long shifts spent on our feet, performing physically demanding tasks, and enduring sleepless nights. However, through the exhaustion and muscle aches, I have discovered the power of self-care and the importance of nurturing my own well-being. By prioritizing rest, exercise, and healthy habits, I have learned to better care for myself so that I can continue to care for others.

Throughout my nursing career, I have always believed in the importance of maintaining a neat appearance, exhibiting clean behaviour, and consistently wearing a smile despite the challenges I faced. These aspects of nursing go far beyond superficialities; they are a testament to the values and principles that define our profession.

The significance of a nurse's neat appearance cannot be overstated. It goes beyond just looking professional; it is a symbol of the meticulous care we provide to our patients. When I put on my uniform, I ensure that every detail is in place - from the neatly pressed fabric to the polished shoes. I do it not just for myself, but for the patients I will be caring for. A tidy appearance brings a sense of comfort and confidence, assuring patients that they are in the hands of a capable and dedicated healthcare professional.

Clean behaviour is equally vital in nursing. It encompasses not only the physical cleanliness of our hands and workspaces but also the purity of our intentions and interactions. I take great pride in upholding the highest ethical standards, treating each patient with respect, empathy, and dignity. I strive to be a source of comfort and reassurance, ensuring that my actions align with the trust that has been placed in me. Clean behaviour is the foundation of trust, and it is through this trust that healing can truly begin.

One of the most remarkable characteristics of nurses is our unwavering smile. Even amid long shifts, demanding situations, and personal challenges, we manage to maintain a genuine smile. Our smiles are not superficial; they reflect the compassion and care we hold within our hearts. A smile can brighten a patient's day, alleviate their fears, and give them the strength to persevere. It is a silent affirmation that they are not alone in their journey towards healing.

The ability to wear a smile consistently is not always easy, but it is a testament to our resilience and passion for our work. We find strength in the knowledge that our efforts, no matter how small, can make a profound impact on someone's life. In the most challenging moments, when we see a glimmer of hope in a patient's eyes or witness the triumph of healing, our smiles become a celebration of those precious victories.

As I reflect on my nursing career, I am reminded of the immense privilege and responsibility we carry. Our commitment to maintaining a neat appearance, clean behaviour, and a consistent smile is a testament to the dedication we have for our patients and our profession. It is a reminder that nursing is not just a job; it is a calling to serve others with compassion and unwavering commitment.

In the face of adversity, I have witnessed the power of a nurse's smile. It can brighten the darkest of days, bring comfort to those in pain, and provide hope when all seems lost. Our neat appearance and clean behaviour are the foundation upon which these smiles are built. They are the outward manifestations of our inner devotion to the art and science of nursing.

As you embark on your own nursing journey, remember the significance of these small yet profound gestures. Embrace the importance of presenting yourself with pride, demonstrating clean behaviour, and sharing your genuine smile with those in your care. In doing so, you will not only uphold the traditions of our noble profession but also leave a lasting impact on the lives of the patients and communities you serve.

Another challenge nurses often face is navigating the complexities of the healthcare system. Balancing the needs of patients with administrative tasks, dealing with insurance companies, and advocating for the best care can be daunting. However, by developing strong communication skills, building relationships with interdisciplinary teams, and staying informed about healthcare policies and protocols, I have found ways to navigate these challenges effectively. Collaboration and teamwork have become the pillars of my professional practice, allowing me to provide the highest level of care to my patients.

In addition to these general challenges, my experience as a plant nurse at the Eveready Battery Factory in Kanu introduced a unique set of obstacles. Within the factory, I encountered incidents such as crushed fingers due to machine blades. Responding swiftly, I provided immediate first aid and ensured the injured workers' stability before their transfer to the hospital. The industrial setting presented its own risks and demands, but being able to make a positive impact on the lives of these workers and advocate for their well-being made the challenges worthwhile. I recommended the implementation of health insurance and worked diligently to ensure its adoption, providing the workers with a safety net for their healthcare needs.

My marriage had a significant impact on my nursing career and trajectory. Being married meant that I had to make certain compromises and adjustments in my professional life. Due to my commitment to maintaining a strong family unit, I chose not to pursue certain job opportunities that I was qualified for. Instead, I prioritized accompanying my husband to various locations where he was posted. Although I willingly made this sacrifice, I want to advise you to carefully consider the implications of marriage on your own ambitions and career aspirations before making a commitment. Looking back, I realize that there were many more achievements I could have attained and goals I could have reached if circumstances had been different. While I am grateful for being there for my children, I encourage you to take a step back and thoroughly evaluate your choice of a life partner before diving in, ensuring that it aligns with your aspirations as a nurse. This will empower you to become the best version of yourself in your nursing journey.

One notable challenge that nurses often face, particularly in Nigeria, is the frequent delay and, at times, refusal of employers to provide timely payments. During my time at the community hospital in Tofa, we experienced a distressing situation where our salaries were withheld for over five months. Such circumstances can disrupt your plans, affect your emotional well-being, and leave you and your family in dire need, even struggling to meet necessities. However, regardless of the challenging circumstances and inconveniences, I urge you to always prioritize your patients. Remember that their well-being should remain your utmost concern.

Yet, amidst the challenges, the joys of nursing are abundant and profound. The feeling of making a difference in someone's life, witnessing a patient's recovery, or simply being there for someone during their most vulnerable moments is incredibly rewarding. The gratitude expressed by patients and their families, the bonds formed with colleagues, and the knowledge that I am part of a profession dedicated to healing and caring bring immeasurable joy and fulfilment.

One of the greatest joys of nursing is the

continuous learning and growth it offers. Nursing is a dynamic field, with advancements in technology, research, and evidence-based practice shaping the way we deliver care. Embracing a lifelong learning mindset has allowed me to stay at the forefront of nursing knowledge and skills, ensuring that I can provide the best care possible. The ability to adapt and evolve in response to new challenges and discoveries has enriched both my professional and personal life.

In closing, the challenges of nursing may be numerous, but the rewards and joys far outweigh them. The privilege of serving others, the profound connections formed with patients and colleagues, and the opportunity for personal growth make this profession a remarkable journey. Through it all, I have learned that nursing requires resilience, compassion, and an unwavering commitment to the well-being of others. It is a calling that demands dedication, but it is also a calling that fills the heart with immeasurable joy and purpose.

REFLECTIVE THOUGHTS

1. Challenges are an inherent part of nursing, but they offer valuable opportunities for personal growth and resilience. Embracing these challenges and finding ways to cope with them is essential for maintaining a fulfilling nursing career.

2. Witnessing the pain and suffering of patients can be emotionally challenging, but it also highlights the importance of empathy and compassion in nursing. Providing comfort and support to patients during their most difficult moments can make a significant impact on their well-being.

3. Physical demands in nursing can be exhausting, but prioritizing self-care is crucial for sustaining one's own health and ability to care for others. Taking time for rest, exercise, and healthy habits helps to maintain physical stamina and overall well-being.

4. Navigating the complexities of the

healthcare system requires effective communication, collaboration, and advocacy skills. Developing strong relationships with interdisciplinary teams and staying informed about healthcare policies and protocols enables nurses to provide the best care possible for their patients.

5. The joys of nursing, such as making a positive difference in someone's life and witnessing patients' recovery, outweigh the challenges. The gratitude expressed by patients and their families, the bonds formed with colleagues, and the sense of purpose in being part of a healing profession bring immense joy and fulfilment.

Actions for Mentoring Future Generation Nurses

1. Encourage aspiring nurses to develop resilience and coping mechanisms to navigate the challenges they may face in their nursing careers. Share personal experiences and strategies for maintaining well-being amidst demanding situations.

2. Emphasize the importance of empathy and compassion in nursing. Mentor future nurses to cultivate these qualities and provide guidance on how to effectively support patients during difficult times.

3. Teach the significance of self-care and the importance of prioritizing one's own well-being. Mentor future nurses on ways to manage physical demands and establish healthy habits that will sustain them throughout their careers.

4. Guide aspiring nurses in developing strong communication and collaboration skills. Help them understand the importance of interdisciplinary teamwork and provide guidance on effective communication

strategies with patients, colleagues, and healthcare administrators.

5. Share personal experiences of the joys and rewards of nursing to inspire and motivate future generations. Encourage them to embrace lifelong learning, stay updated with advancements in healthcare, and continuously seek opportunities for professional growth.

By mentoring and guiding future generations of nurses, we can help them navigate the challenges of the profession while fostering a sense of purpose, resilience, and a commitment to compassionate care.

7

NURSES AS LEADERS

Nursing is not just about providing care; it is also about taking on leadership roles and advocating for change. In this chapter, I discuss my experiences as a nurse leader, highlighting the importance of teamwork, communication, and advocacy in improving patient care and the nursing profession.

Nursing leadership is a powerful force that extends far beyond the realm of providing care. It encompasses the ability to inspire and guide others, drive change, and ultimately improve patient outcomes. Throughout my journey as a nurse leader, I have witnessed first-hand the transformative impact that effective leadership can have in healthcare settings. From my experiences as a head nurse in the general outpatient department (GOPD) of a hospital to my role as a plant nurse in a factory, I have come to understand that leadership is not confined to a title or position—it is a mindset and a catalyst for positive change.

In the GOPD, where I served as the sole nurse responsible for managing the department, I quickly recognized the importance of fostering a culture of collaboration and open communication within the healthcare team. By establishing regular team meetings, I encouraged the sharing of ideas, feedback, and concerns, creating an environment where every team member's voice was valued. This collaborative approach not only enhanced teamwork but also led to tangible improvements in patient outcomes. Together, we implemented innovative strategies to streamline processes, reduce wait times, and enhance the overall patient experience. Through effective leadership, we were able to create a patient-centred environment where care was delivered with excellence and compassion.

But nursing leadership does not stop within the confines of traditional healthcare settings. Nurses possess a unique ability to contribute as leaders in economic development. Their knowledge and expertise can be leveraged to address health-related challenges and promote wellness within communities. By collaborating with policymakers, community leaders, and professionals from various sectors, nurses can actively participate in shaping policies and initiatives that drive economic growth while improving population health.

Nurses excel in interdisciplinary collaboration and teamwork, skills that are highly valuable in the economic realm. Their ability to communicate effectively, build relationships, and work alongside professionals from diverse backgrounds positions them as ideal partners in economic development. By leveraging their holistic perspective and understanding of the social determinants of health, nurses can contribute to cross-sector collaborations that foster innovation and drive economic advancement.

Furthermore, nurses possess a natural inclination toward advocacy, particularly when it comes to social justice and equitable access to healthcare. Their deep understanding of the impact of disparities on individuals and communities empowers them to champion initiatives that promote inclusivity, workforce development, and equal opportunities. Through advocating for policies that ensure healthcare access for underserved populations, supporting education and training programs, and promoting fair labour practices, nurses can make significant contributions to building thriving and sustainable economies.

Being a nurse leader goes beyond simply assuming a position of authority; it requires a commitment to lifelong learning and professional development. Throughout my career, I actively sought out opportunities to enhance my knowledge and skills. Whether through pursuing advanced education, attending conferences, or participating in leadership development programs, these experiences not only broadened my perspective but also equipped me with the tools necessary to lead with confidence and competence. As nurse leaders, we must continually adapt and grow to meet the evolving needs of our patients and the healthcare system.

Reflecting on my journey as a nurse leader, I am humbled by the profound impact that nursing combined with leadership can have. Nurses possess a unique vantage point, as we witness the intimate aspects of patient care while understanding the complexities of healthcare systems. It is this combination of compassion, clinical expertise, and the ability to effect change that positions nurses as natural leaders. We can bridge the gap between the bedside and the boardroom, advocating for patient-centred care and driving improvements in healthcare delivery.

To those aspiring to be nurse leaders, I encourage you to embrace every opportunity to lead, regardless of your position or setting. Leadership is not solely defined by titles or hierarchical structures but by the positive influence you have on others and the lasting impact you make on patient care. Nurture your communication and collaboration skills, as effective leadership relies on fostering open dialogue, active listening, and building strong relationships with colleagues and stakeholders. Seek out mentorship from experienced nurse leaders who can guide and inspire you along your leadership journey. Embrace a mindset of lifelong learning, recognizing that the pursuit of knowledge and ongoing professional development are integral to your growth as a leader.

In the ever-evolving landscape of healthcare, nurse leaders play an instrumental role in shaping the future of nursing and healthcare delivery. We must rise to the challenges we face, champion the needs of our patients, and inspire others to join us in this noble profession. As partners in economic development, nurses contribute to the overall well-being of communities. By advocating for quality healthcare services, influencing policy decisions, and collaborating with other stakeholders, nurses can drive positive change and contribute to sustainable economic growth. Let us continue to lead with compassion, expertise, and a commitment to excellence, creating a brighter future for nursing and the communities we serve.

As a plant nurse in a factory, my responsibilities went beyond traditional healthcare settings, and I quickly realized the importance of nurse leadership in ensuring the well-being and safety of employees. In this unique context, leadership meant not only providing medical care but also advocating for the implementation of measures that would enhance the overall health and safety of the workforce. Taking initiative, I conducted assessments of the factory floor to identify potential hazards and made recommendations for safety installations. These suggestions were not only implemented but also acknowledged as significant contributions to improving workplace safety. By actively engaging with the management team, I played a crucial role in establishing a dispensary within the factory, ensuring that employees received timely medical attention when needed. Additionally, I advocated for employee health insurance, successfully implementing a program that provided financial protection and access to healthcare services for workers and their families. Through these efforts, I witnessed first-hand how nurses can make a substantial impact on the health and well-being of individuals in non-traditional healthcare settings.

One of the defining characteristics of nurse leaders is their ability to navigate and initiate change, even in the face of resistance. Throughout my experiences in both the hospital and factory settings, I encountered various challenges and opposition to change from different stakeholders. However, I firmly believed that change was essential for progress. To overcome these obstacles, I employed effective communication strategies, ensuring that I clearly articulated the rationale behind proposed changes and emphasized the potential benefits for all involved. By fostering trust, building relationships, and actively involving others in the decision-making process, I was able to overcome resistance and gain support for the necessary transformations. These experiences taught me that effective nurse leaders are not afraid to challenge the status quo and advocate for what is in the best interest of their patients, colleagues, and the healthcare system. Through their perseverance and ability to drive change, nurse leaders can shape and improve the healthcare landscape.

In conclusion, nurses' leadership extends beyond traditional healthcare settings, allowing them to make a significant impact on the well-being of individuals in various contexts, including factories and other non-traditional environments. By taking on leadership roles, nurses can advocate for the implementation of measures that prioritize employee health and safety, creating healthier work environments. Furthermore, their ability to navigate and initiate change is an asset in overcoming resistance and driving necessary transformations. Nurse leaders have the capacity to challenge the status quo, advocate for what is best for their patients and colleagues, and positively influence the healthcare system. As we continue to recognize and empower nurses as leaders, their strength in fostering positive change and promoting the well-being of individuals in healthcare and economic settings becomes increasingly evident. Let us embrace the challenges and opportunities that lie ahead, inspiring others to join us on this transformative journey. Together, we can shape a brighter future for nursing, healthcare, and the well-being of the communities we serve.

REFLECTIVE THOUGHTS

1. **The Power of Collaboration:** Reflecting on my experiences as a nurse leader, I recognize the immense value of collaboration within the healthcare team. By fostering an environment of open communication and teamwork, we can achieve improved patient outcomes and enhance the overall quality of care.

2. **Leading Beyond Boundaries:** As a nurse leader, I realized that leadership is not confined to traditional healthcare settings. Whether it was advocating for workplace safety in a factory or initiating positive change in the community, I learned that nurse leaders can make a difference beyond the walls of a hospital.

3. **Overcoming Resistance:** Reflecting on my journey, I encountered resistance when implementing changes. However, through effective communication, building relationships, and showcasing the benefits of proposed changes, I discovered that it is possible to overcome resistance and gain support for necessary transformations.

4. **Lifelong Learning:** Embracing a mindset of continuous learning and professional development is crucial for nurse leaders. Through ongoing education, attending conferences, and seeking mentorship, I realized that staying abreast of advancements in healthcare and leadership practices is vital to becoming an effective and influential nurse leader.

5. **Impacting the Future:** As I reflect on my experiences, I am reminded of the tremendous potential nurse leaders have in shaping the future of nursing. By inspiring and mentoring the next generation of nurses, we can foster a legacy of compassionate, skilled, and visionary healthcare professionals who will continue to drive positive change.

Actions for Mentoring Future Generation Nurses

1. **Lead by Example:** Showcasing strong leadership qualities in your own practice sets a positive example for aspiring nurses. Demonstrate professionalism, empathy, and effective communication skills in your interactions with patients, colleagues, and other healthcare professionals.

2. **Provide Guidance and Support:** Take the time to listen to the concerns and aspirations of aspiring nurses. Offer guidance and support by sharing your own experiences, providing constructive feedback, and helping them navigate challenges they may encounter along their career paths.

3. **Foster a Culture of Learning:** Encourage and facilitate opportunities for continuous learning and professional development. Share resources, recommend relevant workshops or conferences, and emphasize the importance of staying updated with advancements in nursing practice.

4. **Promote Collaboration and Teamwork:**

Emphasize the significance of collaboration and teamwork in healthcare. Encourage aspiring nurses to actively engage with multidisciplinary teams, value different perspectives, and foster effective communication skills.

5. **Advocate for Their Growth:** Act as a mentor and advocate for the growth and advancement of aspiring nurses. Offer guidance on career planning, assist with networking opportunities, and recommend leadership development programs or mentorship initiatives that can further their professional journey.

By taking these actions, you can play a pivotal role in shaping and mentoring the future generation of nurses, empowering them to become compassionate leaders who will continue to advance the nursing profession and make a positive impact on patient care.

8

THE POWER OF RESILIENCE

Resilience is an essential quality for nurses, as it enables us to cope with the challenges we face and continue to provide the best possible care for our patients. In this chapter, I share the lessons I have learned about building resilience and finding strength in difficult times.

Resilience is an essential quality for nurses, as it enables us to cope with the challenges we face and continue to provide the best possible care for our patients. In this chapter, I share the lessons I have learned about building resilience and finding strength in difficult times.

Throughout my nursing career, I have come face to face with countless obstacles, both personal and professional. The demanding nature of the job often includes long shifts, erratic schedules, and witnessing the pain and suffering of patients. It is during these moments that our resilience is tested and can shine through. However, it is important to recognize that resilience is not innate; it is a skill that can be developed and strengthened with time and practice.

One of the first lessons I learned about resilience was the importance of self-care. As nurses, we are driven by a deep desire to care for others, often putting their needs before our own. However, neglecting our physical and emotional well-being can lead to burnout and diminished capacity to provide quality care. Recognizing this, I made it a priority to take care of myself. I carved out time for adequate sleep, ensured I nourished my body with healthy meals, and engaged in activities that brought me joy and relaxation. Whether it was going for a walk-in nature, practicing meditation, or spending quality time with loved ones, these acts of self-care replenished my energy and helped me stay mentally and emotionally strong.

Another crucial aspect of resilience is the ability to adapt to change. Nursing is a dynamic profession that is constantly evolving. From advancements in technology to changes in healthcare policies and evolving patient needs, the ability to embrace change is vital. Remaining open-minded and flexible allowed me to adapt to new situations, acquire new knowledge and skills, and grow both personally and professionally. It is through this adaptability that we can thrive in an ever-changing healthcare landscape.

Resilience also relies on the strength of our support system. The camaraderie and bonds formed with colleagues in the nursing profession are invaluable. During challenging times, we lean on each other for support, share experiences, and offer guidance. The shared understanding and empathy that exist within our nursing community provide solace, inspiration, and the motivation to keep going even when the road seems tough.

Together, we can overcome obstacles and find renewed strength.

Moreover, maintaining a positive mindset is paramount in cultivating resilience. Nursing can be emotionally taxing, and it is easy to become overwhelmed by the suffering we witness. However, by shifting our focus to the positive aspects of our work—the lives we touch, the difference we make—we can find strength and purpose. Celebrating small victories, acknowledging our accomplishments, and finding gratitude in the everyday moments can help sustain our resilience in the face of adversity. It is through optimism and a hopeful outlook that we can continue to make a lasting impact on the lives of our patients.

Lastly, resilience is a skill that can be cultivated and honed over time. Each challenge we encounter provides an opportunity for growth and learning. Reflecting on our experiences, seeking feedback from mentors and colleagues, and continuously striving to improve are essential in becoming stronger and more resilient nurses. Embracing a growth mindset allows us to approach difficulties as opportunities for personal and professional development.

To all aspiring nurses, current nurses, and

those who work alongside nurses, I encourage you to embrace the power of resilience. It is through resilience that we find the courage to face adversity, the strength to overcome obstacles, and the unwavering dedication to provide compassionate care. Remember, even in the darkest of times, the light of resilience will guide you on this noble journey of nursing.

REFLECTIVE THOUGHTS

1. **Self-Reflection:** Take some time to reflect on your own resilience as a nurse. Consider the challenges you have faced and how you have managed to overcome them. Identify the strategies that have worked for you in building resilience and sustaining your well-being. This self-reflection will help you gain a deeper understanding of your own resilience and provide insights into areas where you can further strengthen it.

2. **Evaluate Your Self-Care Routine:** Assess your current self-care practices and determine if there are any areas that need improvement. Are you prioritizing your physical and emotional well-being? Are there any self-care activities that you have neglected? Identify specific actions you can take to enhance your self-care routine and make a commitment to incorporating them into your daily life.

3. **Seek Support and Connection:** Reflect on the support system you have in place, both personally and professionally. Are you actively seeking support from your

colleagues, mentors, or loved ones? Are there opportunities to strengthen your connections within the nursing community? Consider reaching out to others, sharing your experiences, and seeking guidance when needed. Reflect on how you can contribute to fostering a supportive environment for your nursing peers as well.

4. **Embrace Change and Lifelong Learning:** Nursing is a field that is constantly evolving. Reflect on your attitude towards change and how willing you are to adapt to new circumstances. Consider the ways in which you can embrace change and stay updated on advancements in healthcare. Reflect on your commitment to lifelong learning and identify areas where you can further expand your knowledge and skills.

5. **Cultivate a Positive Mindset:** Reflect on your mindset and how it influences your resilience. Are you able to maintain a positive outlook even in challenging situations? Do you celebrate the small victories and find gratitude in your work? Consider how you can cultivate a more positive mindset by focusing

on the positive aspects of your nursing career, practicing gratitude, and finding joy in the difference you make in the lives of your patients. Reflect on specific strategies you can implement to foster a more positive mindset.

By engaging in these reflective actions, you can deepen your understanding of resilience and develop a plan for personal growth and development as a nurse. Remember that resilience is a lifelong journey, and regular self-reflection is essential to continue building and strengthening this vital quality.

Actions for Mentoring Future Generation Nurses

1. **Share Your Knowledge and Experience:** One of the most valuable actions you can take as a mentor is to share your knowledge and experience with the future generation of nurses. Offer guidance and insights based on your own career journey, highlighting both successes and challenges. Be open and approachable, encouraging mentees to ask questions and seek advice whenever needed.

2. **Foster a Supportive Environment:** Create a safe and supportive environment where mentees feel comfortable expressing their thoughts, concerns, and aspirations. Actively listen to their perspectives and validate their experiences. Offer constructive feedback and guidance, while also empowering them to make their own decisions and learn from their own mistakes. Encourage open dialogue and collaboration, promoting a culture of learning and growth.

3. **Encourage Continuous Learning and Professional Development:** Inspire and encourage mentees to pursue lifelong learning

and professional development opportunities. Share information about conferences, workshops, certifications, and advanced education programs that can enhance their skills and broaden their knowledge. Help them identify their areas of interest and guide them towards resources that can support their learning journey.

4. **Provide Networking and Connections:** Introduce mentees to your professional network and help them establish connections within the nursing community. Networking can provide valuable opportunities for mentorship, career advancement, and professional collaborations. Share information about relevant professional organizations, conferences, and online communities where mentees can expand their network and engage with peers in their field.

5. **Serve as a Role Model:** Lead by example and demonstrate the qualities and values you want to instil in the future generation of nurses. Model professionalism, compassion, empathy, and resilience in your own work. Show mentees what it means to be a dedicated and

ethical nurse and inspire them to embody these qualities themselves. Your actions and behaviours can have a profound impact on shaping their professional identity and values.

Remember that mentoring is a reciprocal process, and both mentor and mentee can learn and grow from each other. Be patient, understanding, and adaptable to the unique needs and goals of each mentee. By taking these actions, you can help shape and empower the next generation of nurses, contributing to the growth and advancement of the nursing profession.

EPILOGUE: A LIFE-LONG COMMITMENT

My nursing career came to an end last year at the age of 79. Looking back, I am reminded of the words from Philippians 4:13, "I can do all things through Christ who strengthens me." This verse holds true for anyone striving to make a positive impact and glorify God within their community. It all starts with knowing and believing in God, allowing the rest to fall into place. When you have a worthy dream, hold onto it tightly, remaining focused, prayerful, and conducting research when possible.

Reflecting on the legacy of Florence Nightingale, I recognize the importance of hard work during challenging times. Like Nightingale, I directed my focus to God, enabling me to endure hardships and overcome challenges. I learned from her example of loving people, aspiring to be like Jesus, and extending help to all, not just a select few. To be a nurse with a difference, it is crucial to love every patient and their relatives as if they were our own blood relations. This requires a willingness to learn, humility to listen, and submission to the guidance of experienced authorities, for experience truly is the best teacher. Embracing new knowledge with joy fosters a deeper understanding and facilitates easier learning.

While money is an essential aspect of life, Ecclesiastes 10:19 reminds us that "money answers all things." When I entered the nursing profession, earning money was not an easy endeavour. Instead, I heeded the words of Matthew 5:16, which states, "Your light must shine before people so that they will see the good things you do and praise your father in heaven." My desire to be a nurse with a difference inspired at least two of my close relatives to pursue the same path. The recent burial of one of them in Akwa Ibom State in April 2023 stands as a testimony to the glory of God in heaven. Thus, to be a nurse with a difference, one must pursue their dream with prayer, hard work, and the joy of contributing to the betterment of the profession and humanity, rather than solely focusing on monetary gains.

Throughout my journey, I relied on the support of my family, friends, and colleagues. Without their unwavering support, achieving my dreams would have been impossible. The importance of these support systems cannot be overstated.

As I reflect on the impact of my nursing

career, I offer my final thoughts and words of encouragement to aspiring nurses and those already in the profession. "NURSE." is a heartfelt memoir that delves into the challenges, joys, and rewards of this noble profession. It offers readers a unique and intimate glimpse into the world of nursing, aiming to deepen their understanding of what it truly means to be a nurse and the profound impact nurses have on the lives of others.

This memoir extends an invitation not only to aspiring nurses but also to current nurses, nursing professionals, and those who collaborate with nurses, such as doctors, administrators, and support staff. It serves as a bridge, connecting all individuals involved in the healthcare field, reminding us of the collaborative effort required to provide the best possible care to our patients.

Within the chapters of "NURSE.," I share personal anecdotes that recount the highs and lows of my nursing career. From sleepless nights spent studying during my nursing education to the heart-warming moments of connection with patients, each story serves as a testament to the dedication, resilience, and compassion that nurses bring to their work.

Education and continuous professional development are essential in nursing, given the ever-evolving medical advancements and healthcare practices. By sharing my experiences in pursuing different nursing roles, specializations, and settings, I hope to inspire readers to embrace lifelong learning and explore the abundant opportunities within the nursing profession.

A central theme throughout the memoir is the profound connection nurses forge with their patients. We witness moments of vulnerability, triumph, and loss, becoming a steady presence in the lives of those we care for. Through my stories, I aim to convey the privilege and responsibility that comes with being entrusted with the health and well-being of others.

I also delve into the personal and professional challenges nurses face. The physical demands of long shifts, the emotional toll of witnessing suffering, and the importance of maintaining a healthy work-life balance are all discussed. However, within these challenges, I emphasize the resilience and strength that nurses possess, offering insights into how we can navigate obstacles and continue providing exceptional care.

Furthermore, "NURSE." highlights the critical leadership role that nurses play within the healthcare system. From advocating for patient rights and safety to leading interdisciplinary teams, nurses act as catalysts for positive change. By sharing my own leadership journey, I aim to empower readers to embrace their potential as change agents and advocates for their patients and colleagues.

As the final chapter draws to a close, I reflect on the profound impact nursing has had on my life. It is a lifelong commitment, a calling that has shaped my identity, challenged me to grow, and provided me with a sense of purpose and fulfilment. My hope is that readers will find inspiration and affirmation within these pages, whether they are considering a career in nursing, already part of the profession, or have been touched by the care of a nurse.

In conclusion, "NURSE." is not solely my story; it is a tribute to the countless nurses worldwide who dedicate their lives to healing, caring, and making a difference. It is a celebration of the indomitable spirit that resides within every nurse—the unwavering commitment to serve, the endless capacity for empathy, and the profound impact we have on the lives of others.

May this memoir serve as a guiding light, a source of encouragement, and a reminder that the world needs nurses—dedicated individuals who possess the unique ability to heal not only bodies but also hearts and souls.

ABOUT THE AUTHOR

My name is Mercy Umoh nee George Utuk, and I am the author of "NURSE MERCY." Throughout my nursing career, which spanned many years, I have had the privilege of witnessing the transformative power of nursing and the profound impact it can have on the lives of others.

From a young age, I felt a deep calling to enter the nursing profession. Inspired by the legacy of Florence Nightingale and driven by my desire to make a difference in the lives of others, I embarked on a journey that would shape my identity and purpose.

As I reflect on my career, I am grateful for the countless lives I have touched and the opportunities I have had to bring comfort, healing, and hope to those in need. From the sleepless nights spent studying during my nursing education to the heart-warming moments of connection with patients, each experience has shaped me into the nurse I am today.

Throughout my journey, I have learned the importance of remaining focused, prayerful, and dedicated to my dreams. I have found strength and guidance through my unwavering faith in God, knowing that through Him, all things are possible. This belief has fuelled my commitment to providing exceptional care and serving as an instrument of God's love and compassion.

I have also witnessed the challenges and sacrifices that come with being a nurse. The physical demands of long shifts, the emotional toll of witnessing suffering, and the need to maintain a healthy work-life balance have all tested my resilience. However, within these challenges, I have discovered the unwavering strength and determination that nurses possess. It is this resilience that allows us to navigate obstacles, continue providing exceptional care, and advocate for our patients and colleagues.

Throughout my career, I have embraced the importance of continuous learning and professional development. As medical advancements and healthcare practices evolve, nurses must stay informed and adaptable. I have pursued various nursing roles, specializations, and settings, always seeking to expand my knowledge and skills. Through this ongoing pursuit of knowledge, I have been able to make a more significant impact in the lives of those I serve.

One of the most profound aspects of nursing is

the deep connection we forge with our patients. We become witnesses to their vulnerabilities, triumphs, and losses, often becoming a steady presence in their lives. This privilege and responsibility of being entrusted with their health and well-being is something I hold dear. It is a reminder of the immense impact we can have on the lives of others and the power we possess to bring healing not only to their bodies but also to their hearts and souls.

As I share my personal anecdotes and reflections in "NURSE.," I hope to offer a unique and intimate look into the world of nursing. I aim to inspire aspiring nurses, current nurses, and those who work alongside nurses, to embrace the noble calling of nursing. I want readers to gain a deeper understanding of the incredible impact nurses have on the lives of others and to recognize the collaborative effort required to provide the best possible care to our patients.

This memoir is not just my story; it is a tribute to the countless nurses around the world who dedicate their lives to healing, caring, and making a difference. It is a celebration of the indomitable spirit that resides within every nurse—the unwavering commitment to serve, the endless capacity for empathy, and the profound impact we have on the lives of others.

May "NURSE MERCY." serve as a guiding light, a source of encouragement, and a reminder that the world needs nurses—dedicated individuals who possess the unique ability to heal not only bodies but also hearts and souls.

www.ingramcontent.com/pod-product-compliance
Lightning Source LLC
LaVergne TN
LVHW010608160826
845677LV00013B/3311

* 9 7 8 9 7 8 7 9 9 2 5 3 1 *